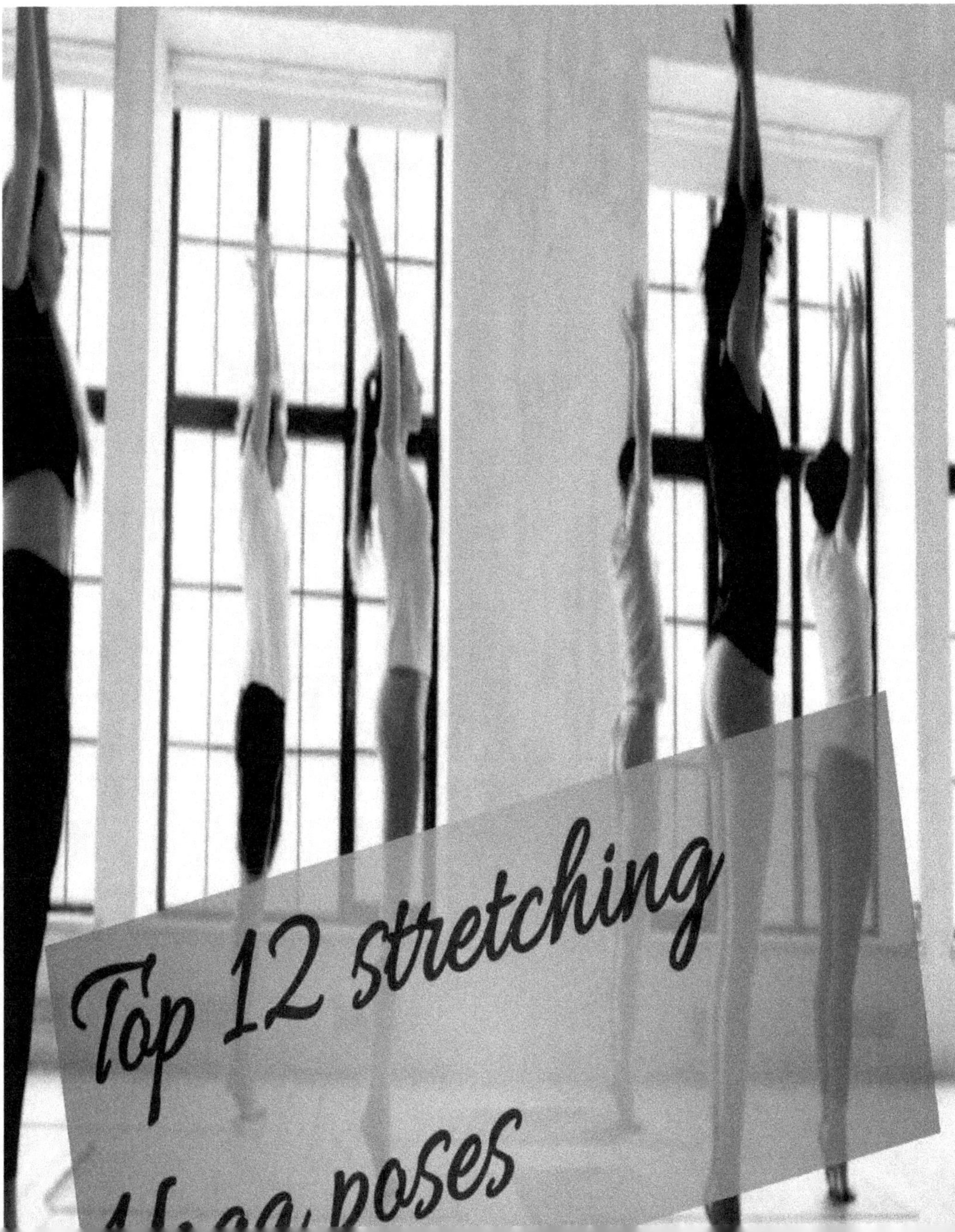
Top 12 stretching
poses

12 Yoga Poses for Health

By

Kundan Sagar

Yoga Introduction

Yoga is primarily a spiritual discipline according to the method of science that focuses on the reconciliation of the mind and body. Yoga is the art of leading a healthy life. The word Yoga is derived from the Indian Sanskrit root word "yuj" which means "to unite". According to the yoga scriptures, the practice of yoga develops the individual consciousness to the universal consciousness which indicates to bring harmony between mind and body, man and nature as well. Living with freedom, health and harmony in all walks of life will be the main aim of yoga practice. It refers to an inner science in which a variety of methods are involved through which a person can realise his unique power. The information about yoga history is found from 2700 BC before Vedic period in ancient India. We get knowledge about the practice of yoga and its literature in Puranas, Vedas, Upanishads, epics and so on.

Meditation can turn fools into sages but unfortunately fools never meditate.

-Swami Vivekanand

Yoga is the journey of the self, to the self, through the self.

-Bhagavad Gita

Yoga is not just an exercise system. Yoga is the science of obliterating the boundaries of Individuality to know the university of one's existence.

-Sadhguru

The meaning of our self is not to be found in its separateness from God and others, but in the ceaseless realisation of Yoga, of union.

-Rabindranath Tagore

History of Yoga

The beginning of practice of yoga is believed to have started with the very dawn of our civilization. The history of yoga is divided into 5 periods : pre-vedic period and vedic period,pre-classic period,classical period(500 BC to 800 AD),post-classic period,modern period (1700 AD to 1900 AD). It was developed by the Indus-Saraswati civilization in northern India over 5000 years ago. The word 'yoga' was firstly mentioned in the oldest sacred texts, the Rig veda. The vedas were the collection of texts containing songs, mantras and rituals to be used by Brahmans, the vedic priests. Lord Shiva is considered the founder of yoga, he is the first yogi who distributed his knowledge to seven sages known as the Saptarishis. They, in turn, spread this knowledge to the seven different directions *covering diverse regions of knowledge that humans can evolve beyond their physical limitations.*

Contents

1. Tips for preparation of yoga

2. Siddhasana

3. Halasana

4. Bhujangasana

5. Tadasana

6. Utkatasana

7. Ustrasana

8. Uttanpadasana

9. Setu Bandhasana

10. Matsyasana

11. Dhruvasana

12. Dhanurasana

13. Balasana

Tips for preparation of Yoga

Before starting to practice yoga, a person has to be careful of many things, only then he knows the full benefits of yoga. Let us look at some rules which are very important from the point of view of yoga;

1. *Prefer a yoga mat for practising yoga.*
2. *Paying attention to the breath is the most important thing, especially when the postures are to be held.*
3. *Learn the basics of breathing for yoga, most important, breathing in and out from your belly. Let your breath be your guide during yoga practice.*

4. *Sit comfortably in any asana posture, move some of your eyeballs to the ground, centre and focus. You can set an intention, goal or prayer for your meditation in the initial time.*

5. *Use a basic level pose and make sure you follow the guidelines of yoga in the right way.*

6. *Always end your yoga by resting your back for about 10 minutes.*

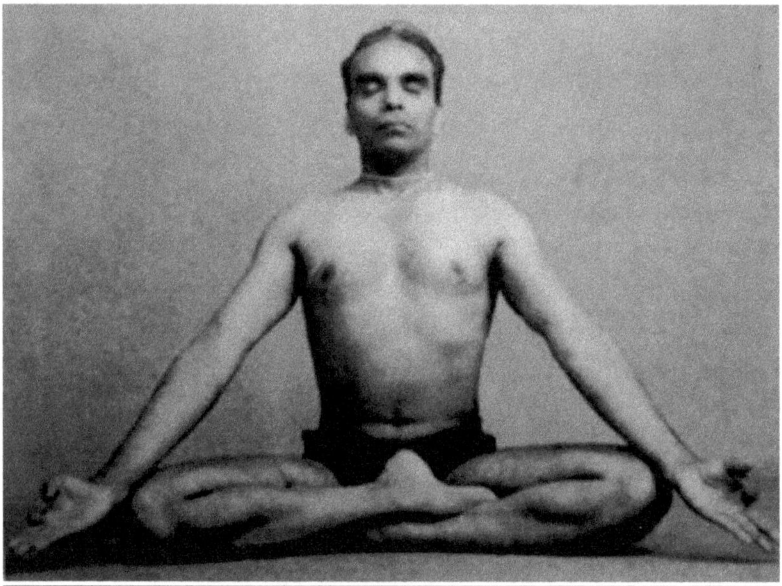

Siddhasana

Siddhasana is one of the oldest asanas, is an ancient seated pose suitable for beginner level yoga and meditation. It is also known as "the accomplished pose" or "perfect pose". The name of this pose comes from two different meanings: Siddha, which means perfect or accomplished and asana which means pose.

Siddhasana is the most suitable pose for Pranayam and Meditation. It strengthens our core, soothes the nervous system, stretches the spine, hips, abductors, knees, and ankles.

__Steps__

1. *Bend the left leg and put the heel on the suture(in the middle of the anus) and fix the heel of the right foot on the sub sacral part.*

2. *The ankle of the right foot should be on the ankle of the left foot. Stay between the toes, thigh and shin of the foot.*

3. *The knee should remain on the ground, both hands should be fixed on the knee in the position of knowledge.*

4. *Keep the spine straight. Close the eyes and concentrate the mind in the middle of the brow.*

Benefits

1. This asana is most suitable for deep meditation.
2. Stretches the hips, knees and ankles.
3. Helps to balance the functions of reproductive organs.
4. Improve the memory and relieve the nervous system.
5. This asana opens up the base and Sacral Chakra.
6. Improves the spinal column and gives a flexible spine.
7. Gives the beginners control over sex urge and sexual functions.
8. Beneficial in the practice of Brahmacharya.

Contradiction

1. *Avoid this pose if you have injuries in spine, hips, knees and ankles.*
2. *Don't do it when having sacral infection and sciatica pain.*

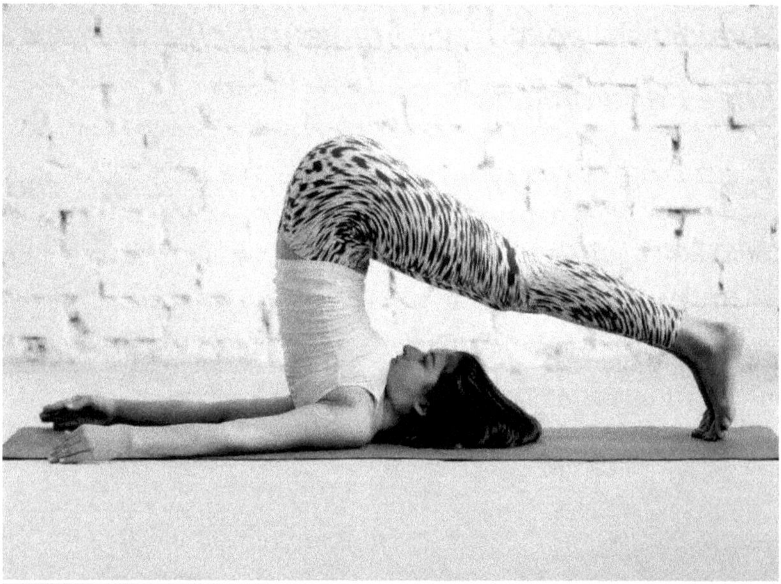

Halasana

The name "halasana" comes from the Sanskrit word 'hala' which means plough and 'asana' which means posture. It's an inverted asana in hatha yoga and modern yoga as exercise, is described and illustrated in 19th century Sritattvanidhi as Lāngalāsana which also means plough pose in Sanskrit. Halsana is also known as plough pose in english. It stretches the spine and stretches, strengthens and tones the back muscles.

Steps

1. First of all, allow yourself to lie down on your back while breathing in.
2. Slowly raise your legs, move your legs behind the head while raising the back as well.
3. Hands can be placed behind the waist for your convenience.
4. Keep your hands on the ground and stay in this position for 30 to 60 seconds.
5. While coming back, keep the feet straight from the knees while pressing the ground with the palms in the same sequence as you had come up.

Benefits

1. This pose calms the mind and reduces stress.
2. It strengthens and stretches the neck, shoulders, back muscles, legs.
3. Make balance in the thyroid gland.
4. Stimulation of the abdominal organs.
5. It enhances the body flexibility & helps to make good posture.

Contradictions

1. Neck, back surgery
2. Hypertension
3. Diarrhoea
4. Menstrual problem in pregnant women

5. Weak digestion

6. High blood pressure

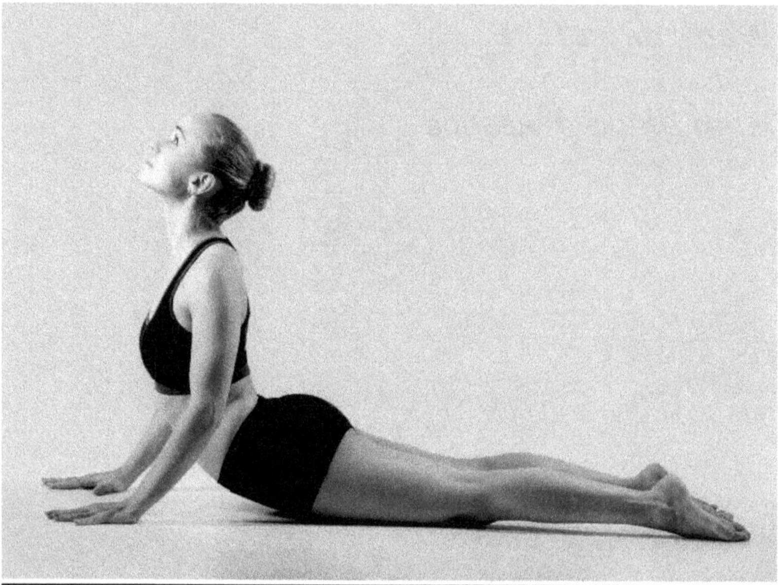

Bhujangasana

Bhujangasana is also known as the "cobra pose" or "cobra stretch", and comes from the name itself bhujanga which means 'cobra' and 'asana' means posture. It's a reclining backbending yoga posture in Hatha yoga and modern yoga as exercise, described in

17th century hatha yoga text Gharendra Samhita. This pose is best for all back and shoulder problems.

Steps

1. Lie down on your stomach keeping the palms of the hands on the ground. Keep the hands on either side of the chest.

2. The elbow should be raised and the arms should be close to the chest.

3. The legs should be straight and claws together, the claws should be resting on the ground with the back stretched.

4. Now breathe in and slowly raise the chest and head, keeping the back part of the navel on the ground while raising the head, behind the neck as far back as you can.

5. Stay yourself in this pose for about 30 to 60 seconds.

<u>Benefits</u>

1. This helps to strengthen the spinal muscles of our body.
2. Stretches the shoulders, abdomen, chest and lungs.
3. Tones the buttock muscles.
4. Opens up the chest and lungs for deep breathing.
5. Stimulation of abdominal organs.
6. Helps to get rid of stress & fatigue.
7. Soothes sciatica.
8. Therapeutic in asthma.

<u>Contradictions</u>

1. Back injury
2. Headache
3. Pregnancy
4. Asthma

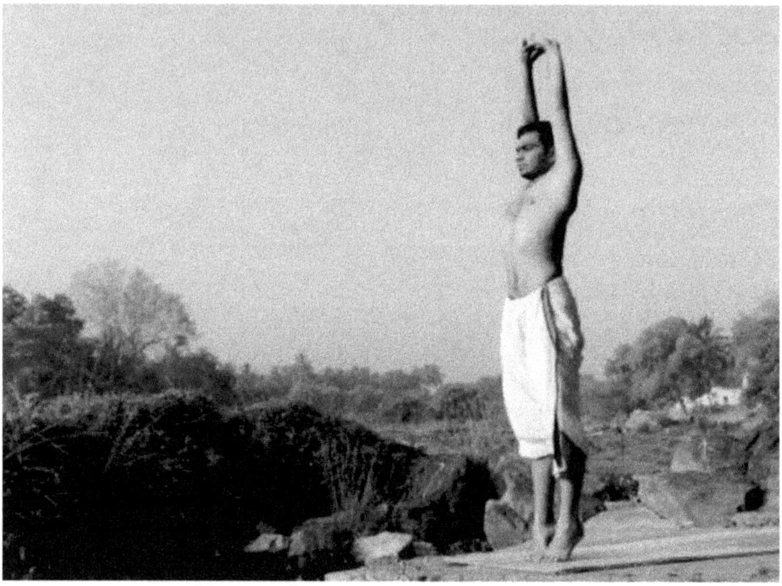

Tadasana

Tadasana comes from the Indian sanskrit word "tādāsana" which means mountain and 'asana' means posture or seat. Basicalliy, this pose is a classic standing yoga posture upon which many other standing yoga poses can be performed. It is also known as "palm tree pose"," mountain pose" or "tree pose". Tadasana helps to improve human body posture, strengthen legs, and increase height.

Steps

1. *Standing as before, raise both the hands from the side while taking a long breath.*
2. *As the hands rise up, the heels of the feet should also be raised.*
3. *The weight of the body will remain on the paws and will be fully taut.*

Benefits

1. *This pose activates the nerves of our entire body.*
2. *Improves body posture and concentration.*

3. Opens up the chest & provides deep breathing to the lungs.
4. Stretches and strengthens thighs, knees, arms and legs.
5. Tones the buttocks and abdomen.
6. Helps to increase height.
7. Relieves sciatica.

Contradictions

1. Insomnia
2. Headache
3. Low blood pressure

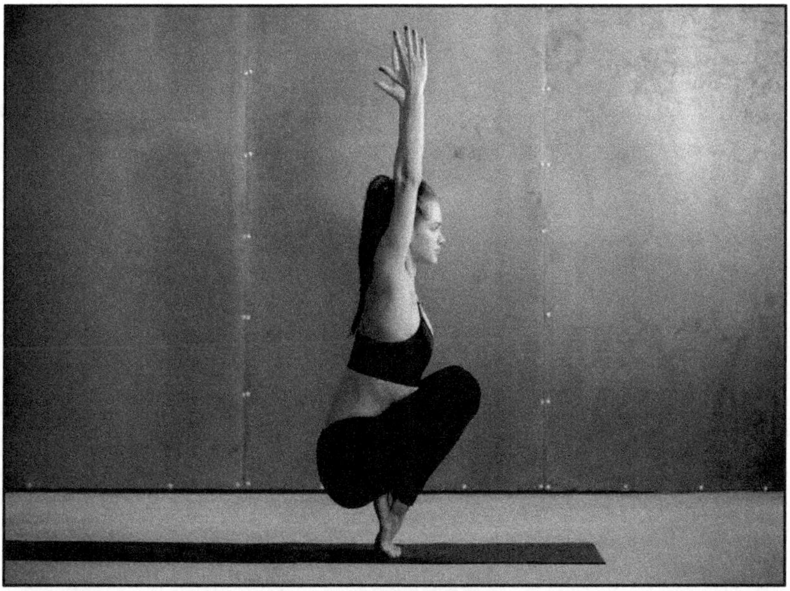

Utkatasana

Utkatasana is a powerful standing yoga posture in modern yoga exercise. The term "utkatasana" meaning powerful or intense position, is commonly known as "chair pose" in English. The purpose of "chair pose" is to strengthen our thighs, helps to stabilise our knees.

Steps

1. Keep the toes of the feet on the ground. Sit with the buttocks resting on the ankles.
2. Keep both hands on the knees parallel to the ankles.

Benefits

1. Strengthens the spine, lower back and gives a better look.
2. Stretches the upper body parts like shoulders, chest, neck.
3. Tones the knees, thighs, legs, ankles and calves.
4. Improves the nervous system of the body.
5. Improves immunity and boosts stamina.
6. Improves balance in the body.

Contradictions

1. Insomnia
2. Headache
3. Low blood pressure
4. Arthritis
5. Back, knee pain

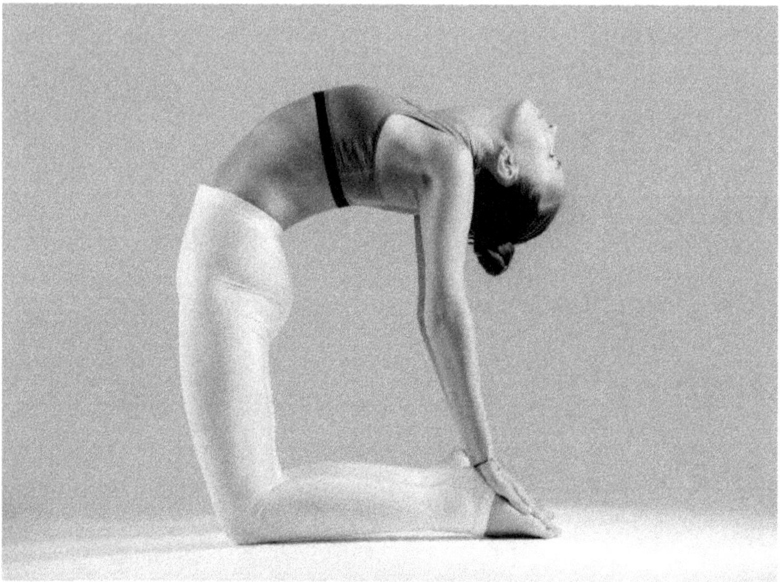

Ustrasana

Ustrasana is kneeling back bending asana in modern yoga as exercise, described in 19th century Sritattvanidhi. The name "Ustrasana" comes from Sanskrit words ustra which means 'camel' and asana means 'posture' or 'seat'. This pose is relieving all kinds of back pain.

Steps

1. Allow yourself to kneel down on the floor with your knees. The thighs should be straight and perpendicular to the floor.
2. Rest your hands on the top of your buttocks, fingers pointing downwards and slightly arch back inwards.
3. Easily lean back and touch and then hold the heels with your hands.
4. Straighten the spine but not strain your neck.
5. Hold this pose for 20 to 30 seconds.

Benefits

1. Stretches and opens the front of the body including shoulders, neck, abdomen and back.

2. *Opens the chest and tones the muscles providing deep breathing.*
3. *Improves digestion.*
4. *Improves flexibility of the spine and posture of the body.*
5. *Strengthens the thighs and knees muscles.*
6. *Relieve back pain.*
7. *Balances the thyroid gland.*
8. *Helps in menstruation.*

<u>Contradictions</u>

1. *Back, neck injury*
2. *Low or high blood pressure.*

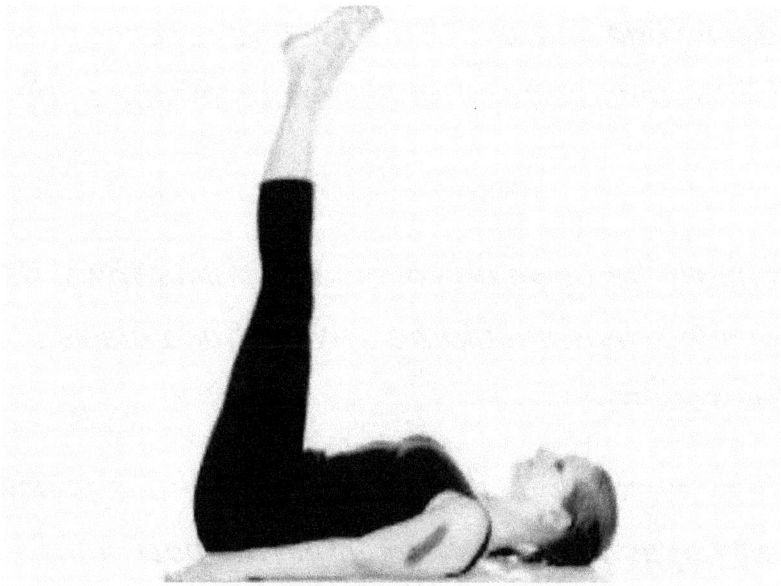

Uttanapadasana

Uttanpadasana, the raised leg pose is a modern yoga pose as exercise, comes from the Indian Sanskrit words "uttana" which means 'intense stretch' and "asana" which means 'posture' described in 19th century Sritattvanidhi and firstly seen in 20th century as modern yoga posture. This pose is regarded as excellent exercise for the lower abs of our body.

<u>Steps</u>

1. *Firstly lie down on your back, palms towards the ground, legs should be straight and claws should be together.*
2. *Now breathe in and slowly raise the legs upward as far as you can. Remain in this position for some time.*
3. *While coming back, slowly keep the feet on the ground below, not with a jerk.*
4. *Take some rest and then do the same action. Repeat this 3 to 6 times.*

Benefits

1. Strengthens the lower back, hips and thighs muscles.
2. Stimulates and strengthens the abdominal organs.
3. Improves the functioning of the digestive system.
4. Increases the blood circulation in our body.
5. Cures the back pain.
6. Helps to reduce the stomach muscles giving 6 pack abs.
7. Improves the functioning of reproductive organs.
8. Beneficial in acidity, constipation, arthritis pain, waist pain and heart problems.

Contradictions

1. Low or high blood pressure
2. Pregnancy
3. Menstruation
4. Slip disc, back pain or spine injury
5. Abdominal surgery

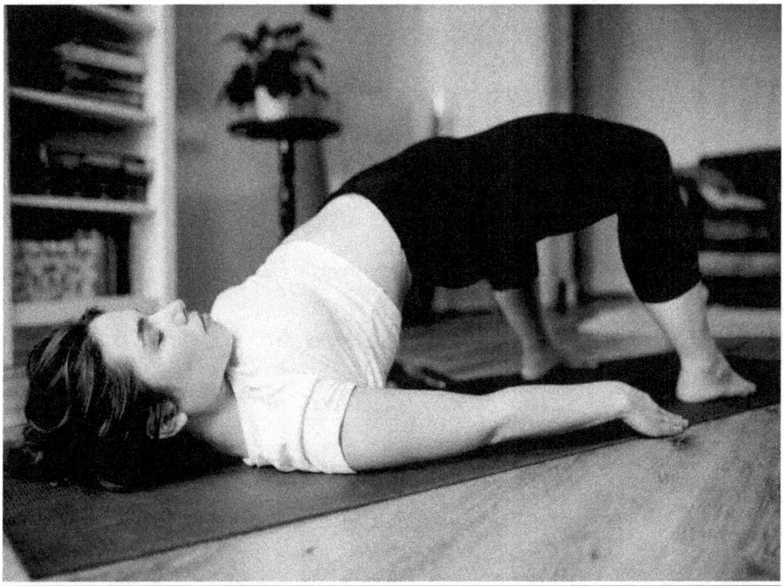

Setu bandhasana

Setu Bandhasana is an inverted backbending yoga posture in hatha yoga and modern yoga as exercise, also known as "bridge pose". The Indian sanskrit words "setu" which means 'bridge' or 'bandha' and "asana" means 'posture' or 'seat' described in 19th century of Sritattvanidhi which is written before 1968. Bridge pose helps to stretch the neck, chest and back muscles and relax our body.

<u>Steps</u>

1. *First, lie down straight on the mat. Keep both knees bent, raise the spine and put both hands under the waist by standing on the elbows.*
2. *Straightens the legs keeping the cut fixed above and breathes easily.*
3. *Remember the shoulders and the head should remain on the ground. The hands shouldn't be removed from the waist.*
4. *Stay in this position for 30 to 60 seconds.*
5. *After staying in this position for some time, rest your buttocks and legs on the ground.*
6. *Repeat the exercise 4-6 times.*

Benefits

1. Gives strength to the spinal muscles of our body.
2. Stretches the neck, chest, back and hips.
3. Calms the brain and helps in anxiety, depression, migraine problems.
4. Tones the buttocks, back and hamstring.
5. Stimulates the abdominal organs, lungs and thyroid glands.
6. Improves blood circulation and digestion.
7. Benefits in asthma, blood pressure and menstruation.

Contradictions

1. Chronic pain or injury in back, shoulders or knees.

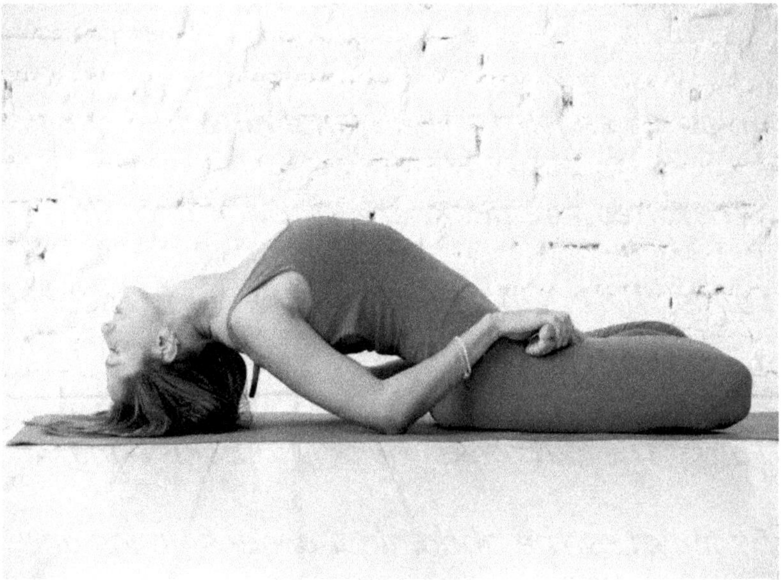

Matsyasana

Matsyasana is also known as "fish pose", a reclining backbending yoga posture in hatha yoga and modern yoga as exercise. According to the Hindu mythology, matsya was actually an incarceration of Lord Vishnu who saved the universe. It is believed that Lord Vishnu incarcerated himself as a fish and helped in transporting all the saints and sages to their safety.

Matsyasana is good for bringing resilience, opening the chest and releasing tension.

Steps

1. *Allow yourself to lie down on your back supporting the body with arms and elbows.*
2. *Now, draw your hands from the slides under the head, bending the hands at the elbows.*
3. *Clasp the opposite elbows and let the hands rest on the mat under the head. Eyes can be kept open or closed as per individual comfort.*
4. *Remain in this position with normal breathing for 30-60 seconds.*
5. *Slowly release the hands and bring them back to the sides and come back to the starting position.*

Benefits

1. Strengthens the muscles of the upper back and neck.
2. Stretches the navel, back, chest and muscles between ribs.
3. Opens the chest, diaphragm for deep breathing and helps in getting rid of all the respiratory problems.
4. Tones the parathyroid, pineal and pituitary glands.
5. Activates the entire nerves of the body and reduces stress and fatigue.
6. Balance the hormones.
7. Daily practice of this pose provides good posture for the body.

8. Helps in constipation, indigestion, anxiety, backache and asthma.

<u>Contradictions</u>

1. High or low blood pressure

2. Pain or injury in back, neck or knee

3. Insomnia

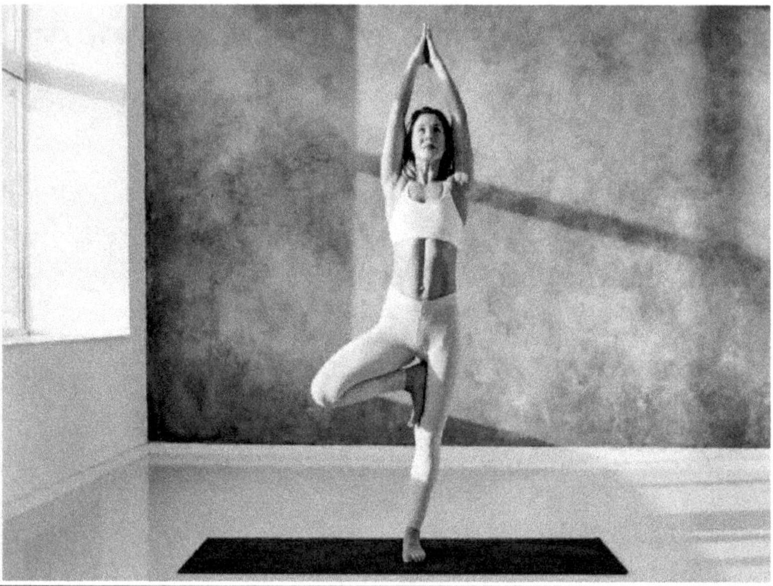

Dhruvasana

Dhruvasāna or durvasana is also a type of standing yoga asana in hatha yoga and modern yoga as exercise. The name of this pose comes from two different meanings "dhruv" which means 'immovable' and asana means 'seat' or 'pose'. Dhruvasana is also commonly known as "tree pose" in english. Steps

1. *Stand straight, lift the right leg and place it on the left thigh in such a way that the toe is facing downwards at the root of the heel.*
2. *Keep both your hands to greet this situation in the position of "Namaskar".*
3. *Stay relaxed and keep your body weight on toes not on your heels with continued deep breathing.*
4. *Remain in this pose for some time and practice in this same way with the other leg.*

Benefits

1. *Improves balance in the body.*
2. *Increases postural and body awareness.*
3. *Stretches the core.*
4. *Opens up the hips and stretches the legs, thighs and shoulders muscles.*

5. Calms the brain and improves confidence & focus.
6. Boost stamina.

Contradictions

1. Chronic knee or hip injury.

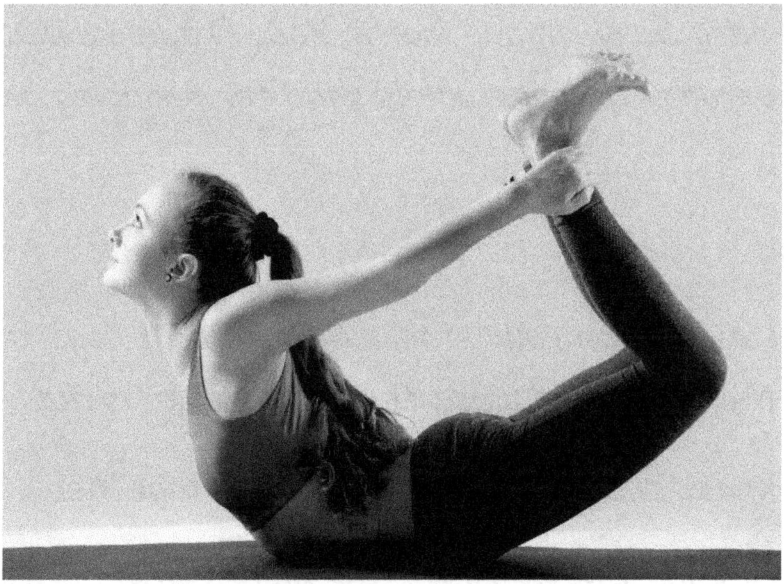

Dhanurasana

Dhanurasana is the one basic yoga pose mentioned in hatha yoga and modern yoga as exercise. It's a traditional level yoga posture originated in the "mediaeval yoga period",comes from Indian sanskrit root words "dhanur" which means 'bow' and "asana" means 'seat' or 'pose'. It's an intermediate level backbending yoga posture, Mediaeval yoga texts like

Gharendra Samhita and Hatha Yoga Pradipika describe this posture. This posture is good for reducing belly fat.

<u>Steps</u>

1. *Lie down on your stomach, bend both legs from the knees and place them on the buttocks.*
2. *Knees and toes should be joined together.*
3. *Holding the feet near the ankles with both the hands, lift up the knees and thighs respectfully while inhaling the breath.*
4. *The arms should be kept straight.*
5. *After the rear part is raised, the upper part of the stomach, chest, cervical head should also be raised.*

6. The navel and surrounding part of the stomach should remain on the ground.

7. Stay in this position for 10 to 30 seconds.

8. Gradually come to the previous position exhaling the breath.

9. Repeat this pose for 3-4 times.

Benefits

1. Opens up hip flexors for better circulation of the blood.

2. Strengthens the back and abdominal muscles & helps to make a flexible spine.

3. Relieve from stress and fatigue.

4. Stretches and tones the legs, hands and chest muscles.

5. Helps in menstruation and kidney disorder.
6. Improves digestion.

Contradictions

1. Pregnancy
2. Low or high blood pressure
3. Injury in neck, back and spine
4. Abdominal diseases

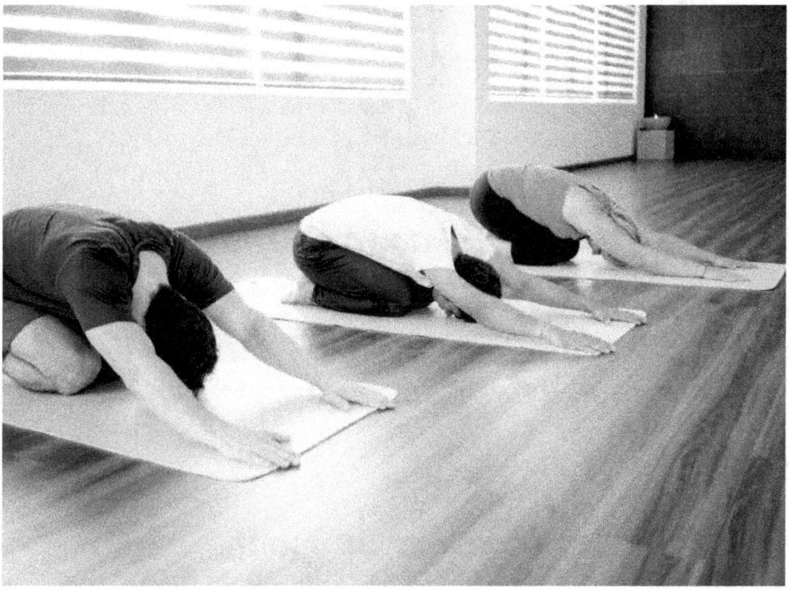

Balasana

Balasana, the child pose is a kneeling posture in modern yoga exercise which relaxes the human body, stretches and lengthens the spine. Balasana is a counter asana for various asanas and is usually practised before and after Sirsasana. The name of this asana comes from two sanskrit words bala, "child" and asana, "posture" or "seat".

Steps

1. Allow yourself to kneel down on the floor with normal breathing.

1. Sit on your legs while touching your big toes together.

2. Keep both knees together or apart.

3. Easily bend forward by allowing the forehead downwards to touch the floor.

4. The arms should be kept alongside your body and palms should be faced up.

5. Remain in this position for 30 to 60 seconds.

6. Gradually come to the previous position placing the palms under your shoulder and slowly inhaling.

Benefits

1. This pose calms the mind and body both and reduces stress, anxiety.
2. Stretches the hips, thighs and ankles.
3. Gives better sleep with strong and steady breathing.
4. Reduces tension in the back, shoulders and chest.
5. Lengthens the spine.
6. Helps in neck, shoulders and lower back pain.
7. Makes supple of internal organs of the body.

Contradictions

1. Pregnancy
2. Diarrhoea

3. Leg or knee injury

***

CPSIA information can be obtained
at www.ICGtesting.com
Printed in the USA
LVHW081817261122
734044LV00013B/576

9 789356 754133